I0441312

I'M GONNA TAKE MY TIME

Malwina Gartner

Premature ejaculation

the source of the problem and how to solve it

© **Copyright for Polish edition by**
  Malwina Gartner & ZloteMysli.pl 2007

© Copyright for English edition by
Malwina Gartner 2014

Original title: Już nie będę taki szybki
Translation from Polish
Agata Majcherczyk 2014

Original title: Już nie będę taki szybki
Translation from Polish
Agata Majcherczyk 2014

Cover photo designed by Freepik.com
and cover design by Malwina Garner

ISBN-13: 978-1505468694
ISBN-10: 1505468698

MalwinaGartner Self-Publishing
All rights reserved.

***
Seattle, 2014

What's inside

About the author

Malwina Gartner is a Polish bestseller writer, that has so far published three guidebooks: "Już nie będę taki szybki" ("I'm gonna take my time: premature ejaculation – the source of the problem and how to solve it"), "Prawdziwy Mężczyzna" ("A Real Man") and "Daj jej orgazm" ("Give her an orgasm"), printed in 2007-2009, and sold in e-book form and paperback on demand, in more than tens of thousands copies in Poland. That means, that during those couple of years the author managed to help countless men and couples. In 2014 her first publication appeared, translated into German (title: Langsam ans Ziel kommen: Vorzeitige Ejakulation – das Problem und die Lösung). Now we are translating the book into yet another language, hoping to bring help to even more foreign readers.

Introduction

Welcome, dear reader, although I realize, that if you decided to buy this mini-guidebook, you must not be in a good mood after all. I have great news for you though. Read this handbook carefully. Start believing, that your problem is not hard to solve, and then try to overcome it, using the information within. I deeply believe you're going to make it. And I'm not trying to make you feel better... because it's not the point. It's actually entirely not... and you don't need that kind of reassurance. You need a solution to your problem. Believe me – You will find it. It will take a little work – and here's the thing – It's going to be much easier if you'll try and talk to your girlfriend. It's always easier to handle things together. But you're able to do it by yourself too, of course. My ex-boyfriend (and the premature ejaculation is not the reason we broke up) thought once, he had a similar issue. And he was right. We solved it together – I was happy and so was he. He felt like a 100% man and we were great together. That's why I know, there is a way out... Finally, I have one more piece of advice to give you. The problem this book refers to, is said to affect 1/3 of the male population. So stop worrying – you're not alone, and what's more, 90% of cases are curable. And remember, that most probably the source of your problem lays in your head. Although you might think otherwise.

Defining the problem

Defining your problem is crucial, so here goes the definition: premature ejaculation (latin eiaculatio praecox) is a male sexual dysfunction, which manifests itself by incapability to control the seed discharge, which makes the partner unable to achieve sexual satisfaction (F52.4 signature in the The International Classification of Diseases (ICD-10) database). That disorder is most commonly related to high sexual tension. In the case of longer sexual abstinence, quick procession of the ejaculation is natural, and doesn't signify a pathological cause, which should be obvious to the man himself, as well as his partner. Sometimes though a premature ejaculation is a constant occurrence, despite frequent intercourses. The reason for this, might be an illness one once suffered from, or other circumstances provoking pain during erection. Fearful anticipation of repetition of these symptoms, during sexual arousal and the awareness of being unable to prolong the intercourse, may lead to an ejaculation without an erection. Making further attempts on the matter is usually unsuccessful, because concentrating on succeeding prevents one from achieving their goal in so called "task-oriented situation". What does that mean to you?

Firstly, there's no one established timeline for an intercourse. You can't say that if an intercourse lasted 5 minutes, the ejaculation that followed was premature, and if it lasted 15 minutes, then everything is just right. It's nonsense. Premature ejaculation is much closely related to the partner achieving satisfaction... - and I use that word with full premeditation, because you should know, that for women, achieving satisfaction is completely different than for men. Not all women achieve an orgasm – that' point a. Not all of them can have a vaginal orgasm – that's point b... and point c – many women achieve their first orgasm late in their twenties. That's why it's possible that when the circumstances are right, your partner can climax in a few minutes, and another time (or a different partner) gets there after a couple dozen minutes or not at all... and you have to realize that. If you forget this simple truth, you will become frustrated and discouraged – and that's a beginning of a really serious problem. You also have to remember, that it's never the same in the bed department... and if the problem occurs only every now and then, you don't have to worry.

Today it's this way, it's gonna be better tomorrow... or even much better. That's how it is now, but darling please wait a couple of minutes, I'll do better in a moment.

And now something for your partner, dear reader. If your boyfriend has a "speeding problem", it obviously affects you both. I'm not trying to place blame here, but what you have to remember, is that you have a great influence over his behavior, so you can help him and yourself at it – because that's what it's all about – that you both feel good and comfortable, right? The worst thing you can do is to make fun of him – men are completely different than us – they get crazy over their manhood. Anyway, what would be your reaction if he told you, your bottom is too big, your breasts too small or that you should lose weigh... it's more or less the same, only multiplied by the complicated and incomprehensible male psyche. It's also important, you don't let him think it's all great, when it isn't. That kind of attitude is the beginning of the end of the two of you.

Your relationship will fail, because after a while it's going to turn out that he is utterly unaware of the problem and happy, while you're frustrated and transferring your sex problems on other aspects of your life. And either you are going to break up, or you'll gonna find yourself a lover, who doesn't have that kind of problem. Either way it's done. Sometimes people behave plain stupid – a woman faking an orgasm is a great example of that. Because, what do you actually get out of faking an orgasm?

Some stats:

- 56% of women sometimes fake orgasms
- 75% of women complain about lowered libido and problems with orgasm achieving.
- 40% of men think women fake orgasms
- 40% of men are not sure, if their partners have real orgasms
- 20% of men deny their women ever faked an orgasm
- 92% of women admit to faking an orgasm at least once

    Source: German studies by E. Frank, C. Anderson, D. Rubinstein,

You think he's happy, he pleased you? I wonder if he would be as happy, if he knew it was all just a disgusting lie, in a moment that you should be in complete harmony like yin and yang. How would you feel if you found out from somebody, he didn't have a good time with you? I understand you can feel ashamed of not ever having an orgasm or having it only after hand stimulation of your clitoris. But there's a solution to that problem too – obviously it's a topic for another publication, but I'm going to advise you to show him with your hand, what needs to be done, and I'm sure it will work out – and you'll both be satisfied.

One more thing – saying "honey, don't come yet, I want to make love to you a while longer" won't do. Such words can create the pressure of a task-oriented situation and may evoke in him the fear of failure… yet you're a woman and you can achieve your goal in a totally different manner.

Do I have that problem?

You know already, that every third, or even every other man shares your problem. But the real question is – do you in fact have an issue like that, or do you just think about it too much? Ejaculation disorders can present themselves in lifelong form, which means they occur from the moment of sexual initiation, or might be acquired, for example as a result of masturbatory activity. Obviously by masturbating, you seek to a fast unload of the sexual tension and by this you create a physiological mechanism of ejaculation within you. During intercourse you are not able to control it, because your organism already remembers a certain behavioral pattern , and does what you tough it to. That's an example of negative training. It all lies in your psychic, and what you have to know, is that 90% of cases have a psychogenic background, and that means, it concerns 9 out of 10 readers of this book. Premature ejaculation, that is an effect of long period of sexual abstinence, or of high sexual tension, is not a problem, moreover it's completely natural (from a physiological point of view). But it may also come about after a period of sexual activity. It may occur occasionally – provoked by certain circumstances. If it happens during every intercourse, it's categorized as a general disorder.

You probably want to know, how to recognize the symptoms? If you do suffer from this condition than:

- The ejaculation happens against your will, and sooner than you'd wish

- You are not able to control the ejaculation reflex.

According to the phase of intercourse during which the premature ejaculation occurred, it can be further divided into:

- Too premature ejaculation (that occurs before the foreplay starts)
- Premature ejaculation (occurring at the beginning of the foreplay, before intercourse)
- Too early ejaculation (in the moment of inserting the penis into the vagina, after a few moves).

You can clearly see now, that it's not that plain and simple, as it seemed. I hope though, that thanks to some advice included above, you are now able to diagnose yourself with the condition... if you actually have it. If it occurs rarely, for instance, while changing sexual partners, you have no reason to worry. Rare sexual encounters or distress after a long break in sexual activity, may produce the problem of premature ejaculation, though in this case it won't last. After achieving stabilization in your sexual life, your problem automatically vanishes. Also, don't read into it, when the premature ejaculation occurs in lack of intimate conditions for the coitus.

Earlier in the book, I said, that premature ejaculation occurs when the satisfaction is not achieved by both partners. I'm gonna say it once more – you're overreacting, if your partner is just unable to achieve orgasm (so called vaginal or G-spot orgasm(1)) during the intercourse. It may also happen, that your partner has an overextended sexual reactivity, which means, the period of time she needs to achieve an orgasm is prolonged. And whatever you do, you will eventually ejaculate. In such circumstances it will be premature no matter what.

(1) Some sexologists distinguish two types of orgasms – vaginal (g-spot) orgasm, and the clitoral orgasm. The latter may be hard to achieve due to rare or none clitoris stimulation – it may be a result of masturbation (often by a water stream).

The Mechanism of ejaculation

Some people say – "first you have to know your enemy, to defeat him." There is certain amount of truth in this, because, to know the essence of your disorder, you should discover how the physiological mechanism of ejaculation works.

The ejaculation of semen is a complex reflex, supervised by different control centers of your nervous system. These are:

- The ejaculatory center on the level of cervical vertebrae C2-C4 of the spinal cord
- Activity on the pudendal nerve
- The sympathetic nervous system on the level of

thoracic vertebrae T9 – T12 of the spinal cord

In a proper physiological ejaculation certain phases can be distinguished. In each of these phases a disorder may occur or one of the phases may not take place at all.

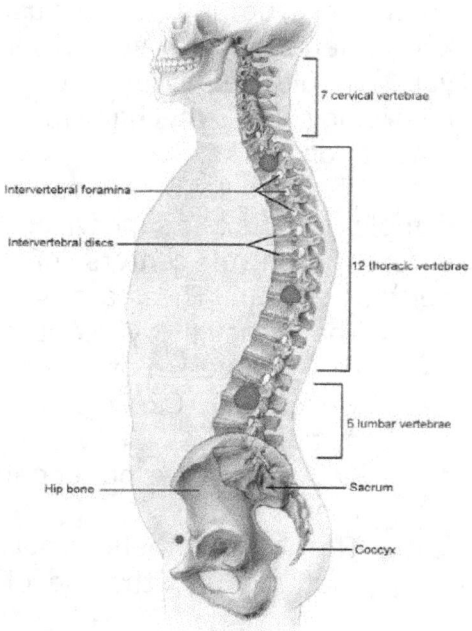

1. First phase is the feeling of upcoming ejaculation, which precedes it by a few seconds. In older men it may not occur or can be prolonged. In the case of premature ejaculation this phase is shortened. This stage is essential to your problem. If you'll learn to intermit it, you're on the right path to succeeding.
2. The second phase of the ejaculation is the feeling of your urethra contracting. It's a great deal stronger in younger men. It is much more vivid in normally lasting intercourses, or in intermitted sexual encounters.
3. It's rather too late now, but you'll find out, that there still is some "chance".
4. Third phase of ejaculation is the feeling of "semen flow"

5. Phase four is the extraction of the semen through the urethra.
6. In young, healthy men it can be very strong, sometimes it may shoot out to distances short of a meter. In older men it may occur without pressure, in a form of a leakage. In hyperactive people it may take form of spermatorrhea.

That's the physiological concept of ejaculation. Its mechanism reminds of domino blocks. When the first one gets turned over, there is no stopping it. The key to success is the first phase – the most important one.

Causes

What are the most common causes of premature ejaculation? In the majority of cases, as I've already mentioned, it has its roots in the psychogenic sphere – that is in your head. It's a well known fact, that sexual actions (like any other actions) may become fixed and connected to the distressed physiological and metabolic processes, so with the ejaculation too. Probably the most important causes for such a disorder are permanently encoded reflexes, that means the repetition of certain activities – a kind of a work out. Often though it's connected to the fast ejaculation training, which is the result of masturbation and the hastiness of the situation it occurs in, the intention of hiding the act of masturbation, the feeling of shame and fear connected to the act, or simple lack of need to control the ejaculation. There might be other causes too, like contacts with casual partners, your partner "rushing" you to come, rare intercourses, irregular sex life. The reason for the premature ejaculation may be an abnormal relations between the man and his partner. It may result in an unusually high level of sexual arousal, connected closely to the attractiveness of the partner, and may induce a task oriented sexual behavior (that is too intense need to satisfy your partner). Negative attitude towards women for example fear of women, of pregnancy, of failing your partner, fear of failure in general, distressed relations between the partners, intermitted intercourses (used as a contraception method without any benefits, and in truth full of flaws), partners faking orgasms, which may be understood as "if she came already, why would I stop myself".

The premature ejaculation may also be caused by organic reasons. For instance: hypersensitivity of the penis glans, too short frenulum of prepuce of penis (constructional cause). Moreover premature ejaculations can also be caused by: urinary tract infections, the prostate infection, diseases such as: diabetes, neuritis, neurological inflammations or even sexually stimulating drugs. It can be surmised, that premature ejaculation problem may be initiated by following conditions:

(From the most common to the most rarely occurring)

- Young age and lovers lack of experience
- Having sex while feeling the pressure to pee
- Physiological reflex, due to masturbation
- Need of fast self-satisfaction

- Rare and irregular sexual encounters
- Frequent changing of partners.
- Lack of trust between partners
- Fear of losing the erection during coitus
- Task oriented behavior
- Awareness of not being able to satisfy your partner
- Medical history
- Having sex under influence (alcohol or narcotics)
- Leading an unhealthy lifestyle (cigarettes, alcohol, narcotics)
- Living under constant stress
- Hypersensitivity of glans
- Too short frenulum
- Inflammations
- Illnesses

Non-medical solutions of the problem

If your problem is of light character and isn't caused by organic factors – and that's the way it is in 9 out of every 10 cases, it's highly probable, you'll find a solution in this chapter. By "light character" I mean a case, that doesn't require a surgical intervention, medicating or specialist consults. Firstly (and that's a must) you have to realize, you will win this battle, because it can be won. And don't beat yourself up about past – think only about the future. Don't let yourself get agitated, don't create fears inside of yourself; sex should bring pleasure, not distress. And that's the way it should be. If you have a steady girlfriend – give her this handbook – you'll go through this faster together. You'll see. If your single, it may be a little more difficult... but also doable. I'm gonna give you an example, so you'll believe me... and though you may find it a bit weird, I count on it, that if I paint such a "male" picture for you, you will get convinced. If you're a car owner, and something is happening to the engine, you're not storing the car in a parking lot, out of fear of what might happen, but you look for the cause, until you find it. You may find out the air filter is clogged, or the spark plugs need to be changed, that's what usually happens. When you find the fault, you fix it and enjoy your car once again. And that's the same as a non-medical resolution of your premature ejaculation problem. What will happen, if you don't succeed to fix it yourself – you ask? Nothing! You just go and see a specialist – a mechanic, who will fix it for you. Am I wrong? And that's the medical way to solve your problem. As you may remember, this chapter will tell you all about the noninvasive ways to take care of your issue. Let's review them than. What's the first thing you should do? You have to be patient. Patience is a necessary condition to the success of your auto-therapy.

Condoms

I completely don't understand, some men reluctance to wear condoms. I get it – you have to put it on, take it off, and be careful so it won't slip – that's understandable. But if you actually diagnosed yourself with premature ejaculation, maybe it's high time to get yourself acquainted with them? At first, let me suggest a solution, that will bring immediate results. There are at least three kinds of condoms on the market, which you should buy, try on and make love in. I'm not going to recommend any special brand, I'm not trying to advertise anything here, but it will serve you well to buy one of those.

Condoms that delay climax

These condoms are exactly the same as others – they prevent pregnancy, protect from AIDS, but also... inside they are padded with benzocaine (2), and that's what matters the most to you.

(2) Benzocaine – a synthetic local anesthetic, for external use Only.

To make sure that wearing these condoms is effective, you have to remember to put them on a little sooner, than you would usually do it. The anesthetic has to take its time to start working. Don't you worry about a thing. When your partner is ready, put the rubber on and wait a while, and the time it takes the agent to star its work – let's say a couple of minutes – you can use to fondle your partner. I don't think she'll mind. When you're inside, don't rush it, you don't have to immediately start to move, just keep doing whatever you did before... you'll get used to the situation and after a moment you can start rejoicing about becoming a great lover. Don't you think about your fear of climaxing... remember, that you have an excellent weapon in your hand (although that might not be accurately described). You can even hide it from your girlfriend (so you have a secret weapon!). After all, these condoms look exactly the same as others, and there's no way your girl will find out about your little secret, if she doesn't see the package. But let's cut to the chase. Don't rush things, and don't make any deep or sudden thrusts... after a while you will feel, that you can make yourself go longer than usual. When you sense things getting heated up... just pause for a moment, but remember to do it early enough. The best solution would be to take your "thing" out and change positions.

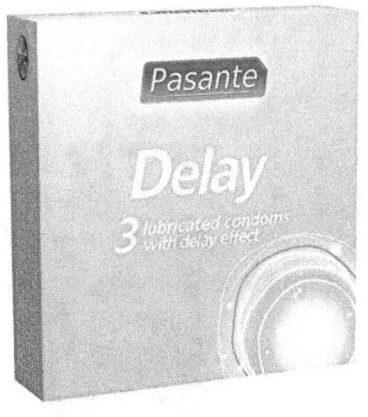

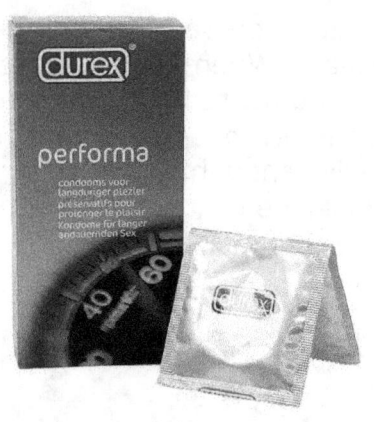

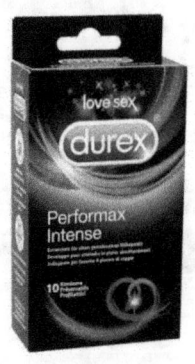

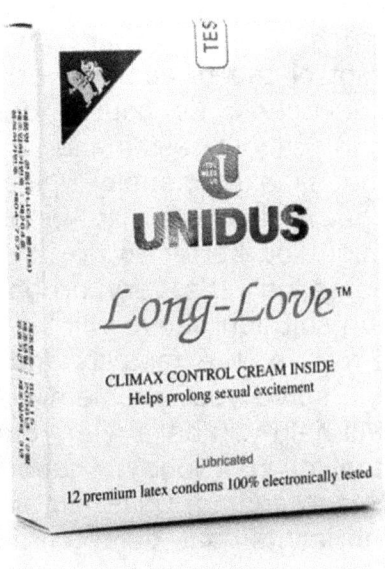

When considering positions –
in your situation you HAVE to
assume one, in which you will be
able to establish control – so all
cowgirl positions are out.
Unfortunately. I say

"unfortunately" because, we – women – like that position very much, because that way we can control the tempo and adjust it to our needs. Of course don't even think about assuming a position that's exceptionally pleasant to you. And what's also important – it might be better to do "it" with the lights off. It's very probable, that the solution above will be the most effective, the fastest, and possibly will solve your problem entirely. It will help you believe in yourself and control your body. that's the way to succeeding. Using ointments and lubricants that delay climax which you can buy in any sex-shop will have the same effect as using said condoms.

One for you – one for her

You have to know, that during one night you are able to achieve an orgasm more than once – supposedly even 9 times– but much depends on temperature. Yet more important than the number of times you can do it, is that each time you can do it longer – and that's for sure. Think of it that way – the first time is for you, you need a moment, maybe a couple or a dozen minutes, and you'll be ready to go again. That time it'll be for her. No doubt you will last longer than the first time. That's obvious an you know it well yourself. You can't just turn to your side and fell asleep, or even worse – start worrying. Show of the knowledge of your physiology. After all, in the time it takes you to regenerate, you can continue the work started earlier – I'm not going to give you any ready-made suggestions, because you are surely able to think of many on your own, and what's more, such that will be most suiting you and your partner. Remember you still have your mouth and hands... women take more time to get aroused than men, but they also get turned off much slower. Warm he up, keep her hot, give yourself a moment, and after that try again.

Masturbatory training

If the premature ejaculation problem you are having is a result of deeply encoded mechanism, which came to being due to masturbation, during which you tried to provoke the ejaculation as quickly as possible, than now, when you are with a girl, your organism just follows the patterns it already knows, even though you're having sex with a woman, not masturbating. To the ejaculation centers in you spinal cord there's no difference. You have to discourage this mechanism from happening. How? just like in homeopathy... by repetition. Now, while you masturbate, and come to the moment when you feel the orgasm approaching, try to slow your rhythm down... if it's necessary – stop completely. And do that as long as you can. This way a new scheme will be created in your head. It's not going to be easy, but the results are what matters the most.

Muscle training

And it actually refers to just one muscle. You have about 500 of those in your body. Women muscles are a bit different than yours, but one of them should interest you a lot. A man can control his ejaculation, if he trains the contractility of pelvic floor muscle, by doing so called Kegel exercises. The Pelvic floor muscle (the dorsal sacrococcygeus muscle to be exact) helps to keep ejaculation in check. How to localize it? From the picture, you can see, that there are a few muscles there, which are more or less connected to each other. That's a fact. Now place your two fingers in the spot between your testicles and anus and tense your muscles, as if you wanted to stop the urine-flow.

The tension you feel is caused by the pelvic floor muscle (when it contracts, your penis and testicles rise slightly). That's the exercise that will help you. To make this part clearer, imagine you're trying to stretch the anal sphincter, but a little bit closer to your penis, because as I mentioned before – all of the muscles are connected with each other in the pelvic floor. You can practice Kegel exercises all the time, not only during erection. You will get satisfying results if you'll follow these rules:

- Do the Kegels three times a day, by rhythmically contracting the pelvic floor muscle, at least 20

times; every contraction should last at least 2 seconds,
- Try to last as long as you can during the last contractions of the series.
- Breathe normally during Kegel exercises; muscles of your thighs and stomach should be relaxed.

After a few weeks of training, you may try to stop the upcoming ejaculation by contracting your pelvic floor muscle in the described manner.

- When you'll learn to do this without an erection, you may start trying it during masturbation,
- After a few weeks of masturbatory training, try to stop the ejaculation completely by using Kegel exercises.

You won't be able to do this at first, but you'll be surprised soon enough. The first effect of your workout, you'll be able to observe, will be the semen flow (a drop or two) without an orgasm. And that's what we're reaching here for. It really works. Kegel training helps women achieve orgasm more easily, and the climaxing becomes much more intense. The pubococcygeus muscle training are recommended by professor Arnold Kegel, in cases of urinary incontinence in women. You may also train by contracting the sphincter just before the ejaculation. Good results can be achieved as well by training in cycles composed of a few warming up contractions, one contraction that lasts 3 seconds, and a few series of fast contractions after that (lasting about 1-2 seconds), followed by relaxation of your muscles after each one.

Applying pressure

It's said to be invented by the Chinese, who very rarely let themselves ejaculate, believing, that every time they do it, they lose a part of their vital life force (sperm is the symbol of life force and Chinese believe it cannot be wasted). That is why they massage the spot between testicles and anus for 5 seconds. It's more or less the same place, I advised you to train by stretching and contracting. This technique stops the arousal. American method "STOP AND GO" is not bad either. The partner caresses the man till he is close to climaxing, and then stops the fondling. She starts again, when the arousal is gone. Pressure can also be applied by squeezing the penis on both sides with your fingers, immediately before the ejaculation, just under the glans. You may do it yourself or you may ask your partner to try it.

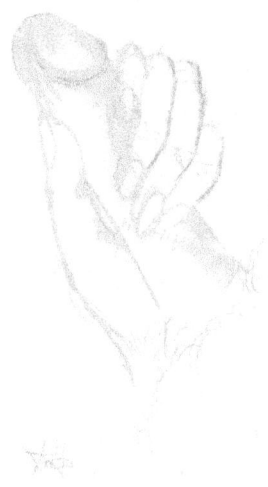

One more advice to your partner now: when you feel him coming, stop him from moving and squeeze his penis where it meets the scrotum for 10 – 30 seconds. After that you may also pull a little of the skin (epidermis) down to help him maintain his erection. Recommended methods of putting pressure on the penis differ, but they are all about the same thing. one of those methods is presented in the picture below. I'm sorry for the quality of it – I never studied fine arts, but I hope this sketch will help you discover where and what you are supposed to put pressure on.

The pelvic thrusts technique

You know a lot now. Before I'll explain the thrusts technique, one more advice. Usually, when it's about to come to an intercourse, both partners are relatively turned on. If you let your partner control the tempo from the beginning, you probably won't be able to last long. It's going to be much easier for you, if you enter your partner slowly, and you'll take your time to get used to the new experience, which will have a very strong influence over you obviously. It will get easier after a moment. The technique is simple. One deep penetration and than 9 shallow ones, than change the rhythm, but so, that every time the sum of thrusts equals 10. 2 deep ones, 8 shallow ones and so one, until you come to 9 deep thrusts and 1 shallow one, and then make all 10 of them deep. When you start feeling the approaching orgasm, stop for a longer while. If necessary, take your penis out of your partners vagina. Meanwhile you can stimulate your partner by touching her vulva with the tip of your penis. When you'll get over the excitement, start again. During the intermissions, you can change positions, but don't stop controlling the environment. Don't be in a hurry. You may also try to think about the disc brakes of your car or motorcycle while making love. Don't tell about it to your partner though. Take that advice. She may not be thrilled. Remember that the deeper and the faster you go the closer you will be to climaxing. This technique is said to be developed from the Taoist concept of stimulating the nerve endings or the transfer areas and is very pleasurable, harmless, interesting and women tend to like it – especially at the beginning of the intercourse, when the rhythm doesn't play such an important role. Breathing techniques are also very important here. The way you breathe during intercourse is crucial, don't hold your breath, breath deeply and calmly, as calm as you can, anyway.

How about a pre-get together workout?

You know you're meeting her today. You're really excited about that, and it's been a while since you've ejaculated. I suggest you should remind yourself about the masturbatory exercises, and by doing that get rid of the excess sexual tension. If you're not overly tensed, it's going to be much easier to take over control. I know you might have heard about anti-depressives or psychotropic pills. It's true, they'll make you go on longer, but they also ruin your organism, you'll feel intoxicated, and moreover – you can become addicted. Alcohol will have a similar effect. On one hand, it lowers the stimulus permeability threshold and indeed you will be able to have sex a while longer. On the other hand, controlling things will be much harder while you are drunk. And you will smell like booze. If you considered marihuana, than firstly – it's illegal, secondly, you can never know what effect will it have on you. No doubt just like alcohol, it will lower your sensitivity to stimulus but you can also start feeling depressed(3). The worst thing you can do is to hold back from intercourse or masturbation, to "gather your strengths" – that attitude will make the controlling harder – after a long period of abstinence a premature ejaculation is nearly a physiological reflex.

(3) Marihuana use can provoke mood swings or anxiety

At the end of this chapter, I want to remind you, that all techniques presented here can be used simultaneously. And the final advice: have you thought about doing "it" by yourself before meeting her? I'm sure it won't hurt – it will reduce the tension, and help a little. Remember, if the method is effective – it's the right method for you – if you'll succeed you will gain self confidence, and that's a step forward.

The medical approach to your problem

If the given methods won't work, you HAVE to consult a sexologist. You don't need another doctors referral for this. What can you expect from a sexologist? Usually, first thing the doctor does is take you history, to make the probable psychogenic cause transparent (the interview usually starts with questions like: when did the disorder first occur? Does it happen every time? How often do you have intercourse? Etc.) Moreover, the doctor can perform an examination of the cremasteric reflex, or the bulbocavernosus reflex (4).

(4) An examination of nerve functions which are in control of your responsiveness.

In justified cases the examination can be expanded.. It may include a neurological examination, or the examination of the pudendal nerve conductibility. The current standard treatment includes pharmacotherapy (treatment with medications). After 4-6 weeks of therapy the intercourse is prolonged average of 2-3 minutes in most cases, and in 1/3 of patients it lasts even 5 minutes longer or more. These medicaments are prescribed by a doctor, and can be used only in recommended doses and under specialists supervision. The doctor prescribes you medicine (for example: clomipramine, fluoksetine), ointments or lubricants that temporarily anesthetize your glans. He can also recommend training methods with your partner involvement. In cases of deeply encoded, incorrect reflexes of ejaculation, injections in the corpus cavernosum of your penis may be prescribed. A man, after being examined and taught the correct protocol, immediately before the intercourse injects himself with prostaglandin into the corpus cavernosum of his penis. This way the erection lasts longer. At the beginning of treatment, the ejaculation will still appear too soon, but the erection will be upheld and the intercourse may be continued. After some time the ejaculation will happen after longer periods. Another way is the Viagra treatment. The effects will be similar, but in that case, after first ejaculation the erection sometimes temporarily decreases, just to spring back again after a moment. In the sphincter muscle training, electrotherapy, physiokinezotherapy and biofeedback can be used. The treatment takes place in a properly equipped specialists office. It takes an average of a dozen sessions, with short intermissions (conducted daily, or 3-4 times a week). Neurotomy is a procedure during which one branch of the nerve is cut. It is recommended in certain cases.

Aiding measures

I don't like the idea of writing about it, but as an author who wants to approach the issue as fully as possible, I have to. There are in existence certain substances, that work quite like the climax delaying protection. Condoms are much more comfortable though, more discrete and moreover protect from pregnancy and some diseases, but other aids exist as well, and I feel obliged to tell you about them. Their prices as well as their brand names differ. They are available in the form of pellets or ointments. These are for instance: "Creams delaying ejaculation for men", "Manly cream of endurance" etc. Examples of products include:

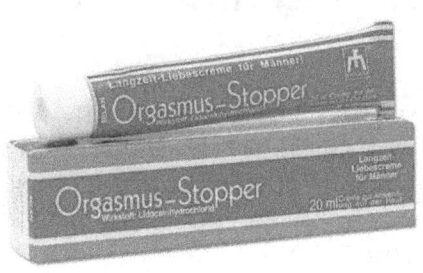

Due to its properties, ointments like that help to prolong the intercourse. They delay men climaxing. The substances within cause partial numbness of the penis and decrease its sensitivity. Underneath, you can see so called erection rings. When putted on, they are supposed to prolong the intercourse by putting pressure on the organ. They come in different varieties, for example for tickling the clitoris (clitoris stimulation). Their purpose is to strengthen the erection. There are also some penis overlays, which apart from delaying the ejaculation are also expected to increase the sensations of the partner.

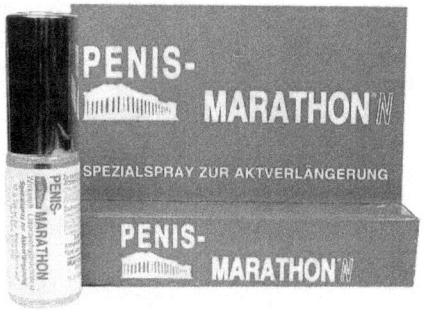

As it comes to pharmacological treatment, you have to remember, that most of the substances that are available to purchase without prescription, that are supposed to resolve the premature ejaculation problem rely on placebo effect. Doctor recommended treatments usually are based on tranquilizing drugs, and unfortunately weaken the organism.

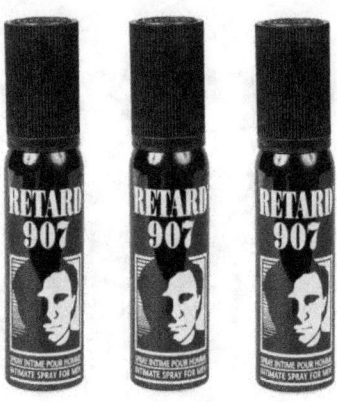

    At the time of this guidebook release in 2007, a completely new drug was introduced in US, named LIF 301, which was said to effectively prevent uncontrollable ejaculation. This was the very first pharmacological substance, thanks to which a man could make love without fear of premature ejaculation, and what's important –

it wasn't based on placebo effect, or anti-depressants.

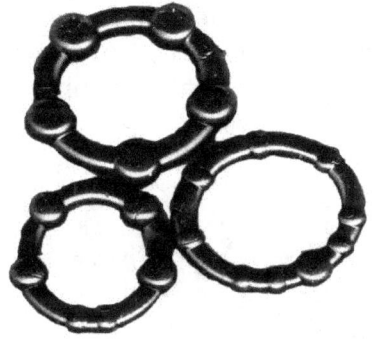

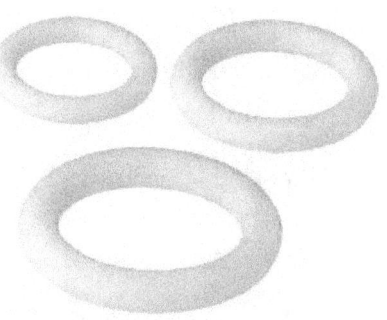

The medicine is supposed to be taken 2 hours before

intercourse, just like the blue pills and… your problems are over! Tests, carried out so far, had showed that this novelty drug does not weaken patients organisms.

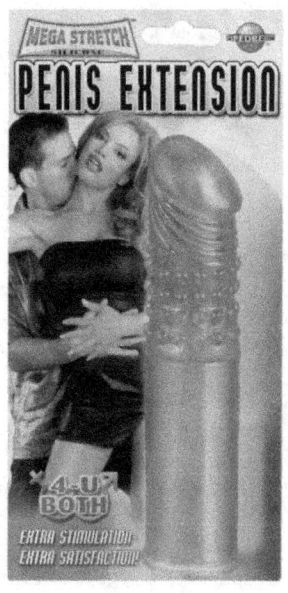

It's available now in pharmacies with prescription. Depending on the producer and the distribution of the medicine, the name may differ. The distinguishing feature is the dapoxetine content.

Additional literature

It's possible, that I didn't meet your expectations, dear reader. After all, I don't have an M.D., and my publication is not a scientific one. If you wish to expand your knowledge (to what I obviously want to encourage you) on the subject, or other subjects of sexual nature, I recommend publications listed below. I'm sure, you are going to find much more solid information than in the handbook you're holding now. I sincerely hope though, that advice, I've given you will help in resolving your problem.

1. Barry W. McCarthy PhD and Michael E. Metz PhD, Coping With Premature Ejaculation: How to Overcome PE, Please Your Partner & Have Great Sex, 2004.
2. David Bexter, Premature Ejaculation Cure: Ultimate Guide To Causes, Symptoms,Treatment & Natural Diet To Overcome All Sexual Problems (Erectile Dysfunction,Impotence,Vaigra alternatives), 2013.
3. Michael Hollinsworth, Premature Ejaculation: The EXACT Steps to Treat What Affects 33% of All Men (Sexual Disfunction, Premature Ejaculation Cure, Last Longer in Bed, Stop Premature Ejaculation, Premature Ejac), 2014.

4. Robert W. Birch Ph.D., A Short Book About Lasting Longer: Step-by-Step Basics for the Management of Premature Ejaculation, 2009.
5. Eve Kingsley, Just F*ck Me! - What Women Want Men to Know About Taking Control in the Bedroom (A Guide for Couples), 2011.
6. Ian Kerner, She Comes First: The Thinking Man's Guide to Pleasuring a Woman, 2010.
7. A.T Emmanuel and Linda Cherry, End Premature Ejaculation, 2013.
8. Ron D. Harris, You cum in 2 minutes... What would you say to the girl?, 2011.
9. Rob Michaels and Dr. Richard R. Howard P.H., Penis Exercises: A Healthy Book for Enlargement, Enhancement, Hardness, & Health, 2013.

10. Helen Singer Kaplan,Singer Kaplan Helen, How To Overcome Premature Ejaculation, 1987.
11. Emmanuele A. Jannini and Chris G. McMahon, Premature Ejaculation, 2011.
12. Michael Castleman, Great Sex: A Man's Guide to the Secret Principles of Total-Body Sex, 2008.
13. K M S Publishing.com, Beating Erectile Dysfunction: Beat Erectile Dysfunction, Stop Premature Ejaculation, Increase Your Sex Drive And Become A Sexual Beast In The Bedroom Once Again!, 2009.
14. David Harris, Premature Ejaculation Elimination - 'Last' up to an hour or more, 2013.
15. Ian Kerner, The Good in Bed Guide to Overcoming Premature Ejaculation, 2010.
16. Darren Marks, Control Premature Ejaculation Hypnosis Session (with Wake Up), 2013.

17.   Andrew Degreat, How joel cure his premature ejaculation without medication, 2012.
18.   John Alan, How To Stop Premature Ejaculation, 2012.
19.   Frederik Lutjens, The Premature Ejaculation Cure: The 12 Step Plan for Ending Premature Ejaculation for Life, 2013.
20.   Alex Ross and Andrew Cameron, How to last longer in bed, 2013.
21.   Michael McClure, Ejaculation Control: Last Hours, Not Minutes!, 2013.
22.   Hypnosis Live, Stop Premature Ejaculation Hypnosis: Make Sex Last Longer, with Hypnosis, (audio-book), 2013.
23.   Kenneth Kee, A Simple Guide to Premature Ejaculation and its Causative Conditions (A Simple Guide to Medical Conditions), 2013.

24. Dr. Andrew Friedman, Stop Premature Ejaculation & Last Longer In Bed, 2012.
25. Michael Carson, The Premature Ejaculation Solution: Effective Strategies & Techniques To Help You Last Longer In Bed Every Time (Premature Ejaculation Cure, Coping with ... Erectile Dysfunction, Last Longer), 2014.
26. Pe: How to Overcome Premature Ejaculation Pe, 1989.
27. Editors of Men's Health, Men's Health Confidential: Last Longer In Bed: Your Guide to Overcoming Premature Ejaculation, 2011.
28. Rasheed Giwa, How to Cure Quick Ejaculation Without Drugs, 2012.
29. Chris Buchanan, 5 Great Ways To Last Longer In The Bedroom, 2013.

30.   Jacob C. Williams, Premature Ejaculation - New Hope for an Old Problem, 2005.

31.   Janet Hall, Stop Premature Ejaculation Now - Overcome and Cure Sexual Related Issues (No More Premature Ejaculation - Dr Janet Hall's - You Can Have Sensational Sex Series), 2013.

32.   Darren Marks, Overcome Premature Ejaculation: Take Control of Your Mind and Body and Become a Great Lover, (audio-book), 2009.

33.   Conor Patrick JR and Lee Neale, Immature Ejaculation, 2013.

34.   Vincent Atwell, Sexcess: Flip The "Sex Switch" & Stop Premature Ejaculation Permanently, Increase Sexual Stamina & Last Longer In Bed In Just 2 Easy Steps, 2011.

35.   Tim James, Stopping Premature Ejaculation: Volume 1 The Guide, 2011.

36.   Jason Whitten, Premature Ejaculation: Treatment, Cures and Preventing Premature Ejaculation, 2012.
37.   Joanne Ferro and Joan Goldberg, Premature Ejaculation (Sexual Healing Guides Book 3), 2012.
38.   Anthony Ekanem, Bedroom Secrets For Men: How To Stop Pre-Mature Ejaculation Naturally and Permanently, 2014.

Final word

I guess that's all the advice, I can now give you. I know the situation you're in is not easy, but you have to remember, that you're a man, and that's the reason it's so hard on you. You take it all too personally – which is typical to your "kind". That's why your problem appears to be even worse. The methods I described, that help prolong the intercourse are usually very effective, and I'm sure they will help, and if not... you'll have to consult a specialist, but you probably know that already. Maybe this guidebook will be the impulse to get you to go and see a doctor, if the means described won't do. If that's what happens – my handbook did it's work. If there is a real problem – it has to be taken care of, not to provoke other complications, usually of psychological nature. And lastly – don't avoid sexual contacts! It's the worst mistake you could make! The more, the better – remember that – the more you'll make love, the better results you will get. Good luck!

Malwina Gartner

malwina-gartner@o2.pl

www.ingramcontent.com/pod-product-compliance
Lightning Source LLC
Chambersburg PA
CBHW060643290526
45793CB00001B/373